Introduction

The Ketogenic Diet, originally known as the Ketogenic Therapy, was created in 1923 as a treatment for epilepsy by Dr. Russell Wilder. It was popular in the 1920s until it was abandoned in favor of anticonvulsant drugs.

Today, the Ketogenic diet, or the Keto diet as it is more commonly known, has made a return to mainstream popularity as an effective weight loss diet. Essentially, the Keto Diet is a high-fat and low-carb diet that may help in losing weight and providing more energy, among other benefits.

The sudden and drastic reduction of carbs puts the body into a metabolic state called Ketosis, a state in which the body becomes efficient at burning fat for energy. Additionally, this process produces Ketones, which are not only used as energy for the brain, but have also been shown to curb appetite, a factor which may also help in losing weight by reducing food consumption.

This book is for people who would like to discover more about the Ketogenic diet, but are worried that they may get things wrong. The information in this book is not meant to replace any medication or treatment regimen that you may already have. Please do not proceed with this diet without discussing the risks and rewards with your healthcare provider, especially if you have an underlying medical condition, like diabetes or hypertension.

What are you going to learn on this journey?

- **A little background on the Ketogenic diet.** And don't worry! We're not going to be too science-heavy. We'll just cover the basics before proceeding with the other chapters.

- **The many benefits of the keto diet.** You may be surprised to know that the Ketogenic diet could help a lot of common conditions, including high blood pressure, high levels of bad cholesterol, and even diabetes!

- **Most common misconceptions about the diet.** Don't believe everything you see online! Even people who claim to have "tried and tested" the diet, may, in reality, have just carelessly cut down on their carbs and binged on fats! Be informed – the right way!

- **A step-by-step Guide on How to Start the Keto Diet.** How are you going to start your Ketogenic diet? In this section, we'll give you a blow by blow account of how to achieve ketosis to enable you to lose all that excess weight.

- **Detailed Explanation regarding if Keto is for you or not for you.** As much as you want to enter the keto regimen, it might be that it's not for you. To better assess yourself, we have prepared a detailed chapter to determine if keto is right for you or if you need to look for another dietary routine.

- **Shopping List.** Guess what? We have also prepared, for you, a list of foods to eat, foods to avoid, and drinks that are just right. With all these choices, you'll have a lot of ingredients to experiment with to create tasty, safe, and healthy recipes.

- **Practical Tips.** At the end of this book, you will be given many practical tips about the process of reaching ketosis, about checking when you're in ketosis, and also about determining your long-term goal after the keto diet.

So if you're ready, let's proceed to the journey!

Contents

Practical Tips When It Comes to Ketogenic Diet

Simple Keto Recipes

Conclusion

Chapter 1

The Ketogenic Diet at a Glance

In this introductory chapter, we will have a brief explanation about what the Ketogenic diet is. Don't worry! We'll also have detailed discussions as we progress in the book. This chapter just aims to "stretch" our brain muscles to absorb what's to come.

Where Do We Get Our Energy?

To fully understand the Ketogenic diet, we need to appreciate the basics of digestion.

You see, for us to live and thrive, we need nutrition. We eat food and break down its components into smaller nutrients that will eventually enter our cells. We have three main sources of these nutrients: carbohydrates, proteins, and fats.

Among the three, the body's preferred source is carbohydrates. This is because the calories in carbohydrates are easier to break down compared to the calories in the proteins and fats.

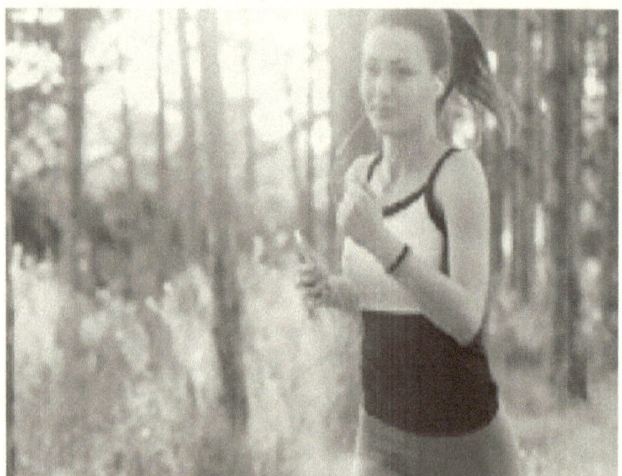

Now, here's the problem:

When we eat too many carbohydrates, some of the calories will be unused. These unused carbs will turn into glycogen or fats, which will then appear as unwanted flab on our tummies and extra cushions on our love handles.

 According to the Ketogenic diet, these fats cannot be shed unless your body consumes them. One way to consume them is to cut down on your carbohydrate intake and allow your body to instead, use the calories from your stored fat as energy.

 This is where the Ketogenic diet enters.

What is the Ketogenic Diet?

The Ketogenic diet is a diet that releases substances called ketones. These ketones are produced when our body uses energy from stored fats instead of the typical sugar or carbohydrates. But this can't happen through a casual cutting down of carbs. You need to take most of your nutrients from fats and proteins and *extremely* limit your carb intake.

 If you do that, your body will have no choice but to get its energy from the excess fats that you have, and the result is: a rapid and real weight loss.

Key Takeaways

The Ketogenic diet is a low-carb, high-fat diet. It's highly restrictive, and that's why people who opt for this regimen should prepare physically and mentally before embarking on this journey.

Chapter 2

The Benefits of Ketogenic Diet

Now that you have a bird's eye view of what the Ketogenic diet is, let's move on to what could be one of the most interesting parts: discussing its benefits.

Aside from the fact that the Ketogenic diet will help you lose weight, you'll also receive an additional variety of benefits.

It Helps in Treating Epilepsy in Children

If we want to talk about proven keto benefits, then this is definitely one of them: it helps treat epilepsy in children. In fact, the Ketogenic diet is so effective that doctors have been using it since the 1920s!

Looking at the figures, you'll be surprised to know that the keto diet can decrease the number of seizures experienced by epileptic children by half! Additionally, according to Everyday Health, 10 to 15 % of those who used this diet regimen become seizure free. Finally, it can also help children decrease the dose of their seizure drugs.

Is keto also effective in treating epilepsy in adults?

Unfortunately, it's not highly recommended for epileptic adults because the strict dietary requirement makes it hard for adults to maintain it. However, there are studies suggesting that it may still help.

A study using adult subjects showed that the participants who managed to use the diet significantly reduced the number of seizures experienced and that 7% became seizure-free after maintaining the keto diet for 4 years.

It Helps You Lose Weight

This is the reason that most people decide to switch to the Ketogenic diet routine: they want to be slim and trim and shed all that excess weight which is ruining their lives. And the Ketogenic diet can help you lose all that weight in more ways than one. We will discuss all those ways in this section.

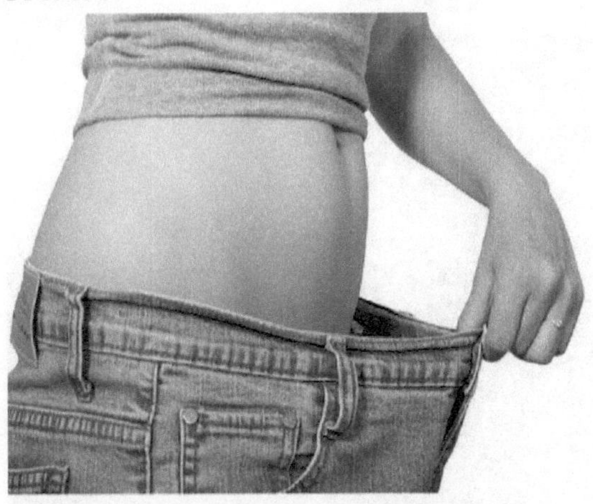

The Ketogenic Diet Helps Reduce Your Appetite

The biggest hurdle most people experience when they go on a normal weight reducing diet, is that dreadful feeling of hunger and deprivation. You are eating less than before, so it's not surprising that you crave more food. The more you continue to resist your cravings, the more you'll feel deprived. Sooner or later, you might just give up on dieting altogether.

You'll be happy to know that this is an entirely different experience. The Ketogenic diet actually helps to curb your appetite, because, the more you take your calories from fats and proteins, the less you'll crave other food.

The Keto Diet Helps You Lose a Lot at First

While the heading above makes it seem like you'll only lose weight in the beginning of the diet, don't fret. What we mean by the statement: *keto helps you lose a lot of weight at first*, is that weight loss is very noticeable in the beginning of the diet and then tails off.

This is both a good thing and something that you need to be careful about. According to experts, the Ketogenic diet makes you lose water, that's why you lose a lot of weight rapidly in the beginning of the process, particularly in the first and second week. So don't become discouraged; the weight loss may tail off after the initial dramatic effect, but the fat will keep being used and your overall weight will continue to drop, just more slowly.

It May Help Treat Acne

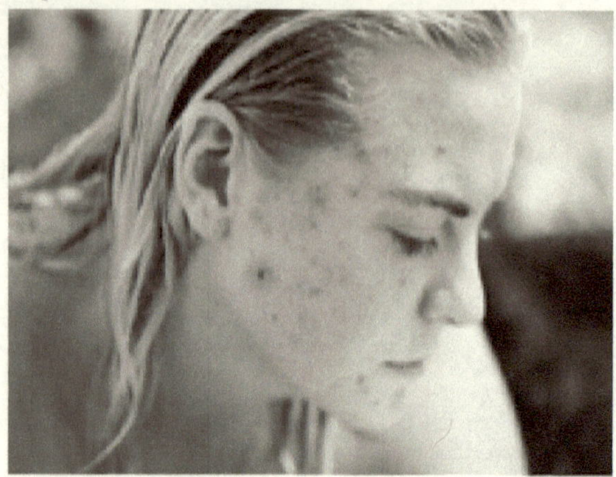

As crazy as it sounds, the Ketogenic diet could actually help to clear your skin of those annoying and unsightly spots and pimples. !

According to Medical News Today, a diet high in "processed and refined" sugar may

    a. Affect the number of bacteria in the gut, and
    b. Fluctuate the level of blood glucose.

As both of these things affect skin health, one can only conclude that cutting out sugar from the diet would eliminate spots and pimples. And one study concluded that a low carb diet- in particular- reduced acne symptoms for some people.

It Could Help with Brain Health

Brain training is big business. A lot of people are paying just to increase their chances of staving off possible brain-related diseases such as Alzheimer's. Right now, the most popular method of boosting one's brain appears to be through brain-training apps.

However, people should know that there are other ways to boost our brain health – like the Ketogenic diet.

Hold up! We're not saying that it's now medically proven, because more studies are still needed in order to claim that. But you cannot discount the fact that there is at least one study suggesting that the ketones produced once a person is in the state of ketosis actually help protect our neurons or brain cells.

At this point, we haven't really talked about ketosis yet, but we will later. For now, it's enough that you know that when you are on the Ketogenic diet, you will release some ketones! Ketones are chemicals made by our liver when we don't have enough sugar. In other words, instead of relying on glucose for energy, we will rely on ketones, instead. It's also interesting to note that ketones are basically acid, which is why you may become acidic when you're on the keto diet.

It Might Help With Type 2 Diabetes

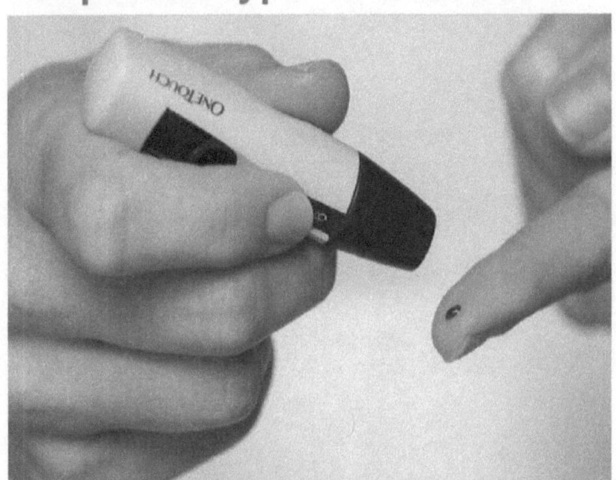

Here's one possible benefit that, though ironic, is still worth discussing: the Ketogenic diet may possibly help with Type 2 diabetes.

Diabetes is a condition wherein sugar cannot be properly "digested" by our cells. Unable to enter the cell, the sugar remains in the blood, resulting in the telltale sign of high glucose level. In their desire to lower down their blood glucose level, people who have diabetes become very conscious of their diet – often forgoing foods like cakes, ice cream, sodas, and even rice, since as well as the straight sugar content, the carbs in these foodstuffs are also converted into glucose.

This proactive reduction in carb intake is quite similar to that which someone who is on the Ketogenic diet is doing. The only difference is that on the keto diet, you will rely *heavily* on fats.

It's quite ironic, given that the keto diet reduces sugar and carb intake, that people who have diabetes are cautioned against this diet. It is, however, understandable, because the drastic decrease in the blood sugar level may cause them to experience hypoglycemia.

Hypoglycemia is the medical term for having an abnormally low blood glucose level and this is not good even for diabetics.

Despite this, the Ketogenic diet is still said to be beneficial for people with Type 2 diabetes, so long as they do it with extreme caution and with the guidance of their doctor.

It Could Improve Your Blood Pressure

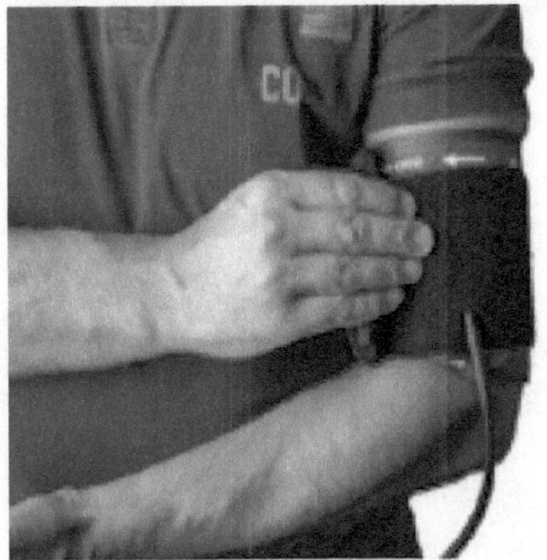

How many people have problems when it comes to their blood pressure? A lot, right?

Because they understand the Ketogenic diet as a diet that is high in fat, many people steer clear of it. After all, too much fat will cause their blood pressure to rise.

Well, they could be wrong.

According to Ruled Me, there was a study suggesting that the Ketogenic diet may just be the "solution" for hypertension.

In that particular study, participating women tried 4 diet regimens – one of which was the Ketogenic diet. After a year of religiously following their designated diet, the researchers checked their blood pressure as well as other parameters that demonstrated the health of their hearts, such as body mass, triglyceride levels, and bad cholesterol levels.

Guess what?

The women in the low-carbohydrate group had the best results. Not only did they show lower body mass, triglycerides, and bad cholesterol, they also significantly lowered their blood pressure! Their systolic pressure was lowered by 7.6 mmhg – twice that of the rest of the participants on the other diets.

But as with the case in Type 2 Diabetes, people who have high blood pressure should not be too quick to follow this diet solely for the reason of managing their hypertension. Aside from making sure that they are proceeding carefully with the diet, they should also consult their doctor before they start. .

It can Help in Treating PCOS and Perhaps Even Infertility

PCOS or Polycystic Ovarian Syndrome is a common condition amongst women. It is also a common cause of infertility. To briefly discuss PCOS: it's a condition wherein the woman produces more male hormones than normal. This results in symptoms like the growth of chest-hair, loss of libido or sex drive, and mood swings. The interesting thing is PCOS is linked to a woman's insulin level, which could be lowered down by the keto diet.

In one study, 5 women who were overweight followed a strict Ketogenic diet with just 20 grams of carbohydrates per day. After 24 weeks of being on the diet, the women showed the following results:

- Average weight loss of 12%
- Decreased free testosterone level by 22%
- Decreased level of fasting insulin

In an even more interesting turn of events, two of the women fell pregnant!

While it's too soon to tell whether the Ketogenic diet really helps in PCOS and infertility management, this study suggests strongly that it may well do so. And we'll hold onto that possibility until other studies about it emerge.

It Helps Manage Cholesterol

You may be surprised to know that a diet that is high in fat can actually help you maintain a healthy cholesterol level. When we say "healthy" we're referring to a low level of LDL and a high level of HDL.

LDL, or low-density lipoprotein, is also called bad cholesterol, since an increase in its level is linked with different cardiovascular diseases. On the other hand, HDL or high-density lipoprotein is considered to be 'good' cholesterol.

One way to check if you're managing your cholesterol levels adequately, is to take the total amount of your cholesterol and divide it by the amount of HDL in your body. If you get a result of 3.5 or lower, then you can rest easy that you have a good cholesterol level.

Some studies indicate that being on the Ketogenic diet may help to promote healthy cholesterol. .

As we discussed with regards to diabetes, hypertension, and even PCOS, the relationship between cholesterol and the keto diet is not definitively proven. . Some people who chose the keto diet experienced a surge not just in their total cholesterol, but also in their LDL. This is essentially bad. However, we can't discount the results recorded by other people who developed a good ratio between their total cholesterol and their HDL after being on the keto diet.

As always, if you have problems with your cholesterol and you would like to resolve it with the keto diet, the best course of action is to talk to your physician. You don't want to dive straight into this routine without knowing which fat is good or bad for you.

Key Takeaways

A lot of studies are already centered on knowing if the Ketogenic diet is helpful in various conditions like diabetes, high levels of bad cholesterol, PCOS, and hypertension. Although more studies are needed to prove that the keto diet may assist in medical conditions, the keto diet is most definitely proving to be very promising in the case of people who would like to shed their excess pounds!

Chapter 3

Ketogenic Diet Misconceptions Debunked

With the Keto diet being discussed in the news, health forums or in gym conversations, you probably want to try it as soon as possible. *Especially* after reading about its numerous benefits! But wait up –as we have emphasized in the past chapter, you can't just leap without looking. You need to know which things about Keto are true, and which ones aren't.

 Here are some of the biggest misconceptions about the Ketogenic diet.

You have a license to eat any kind of fat, as much as you want

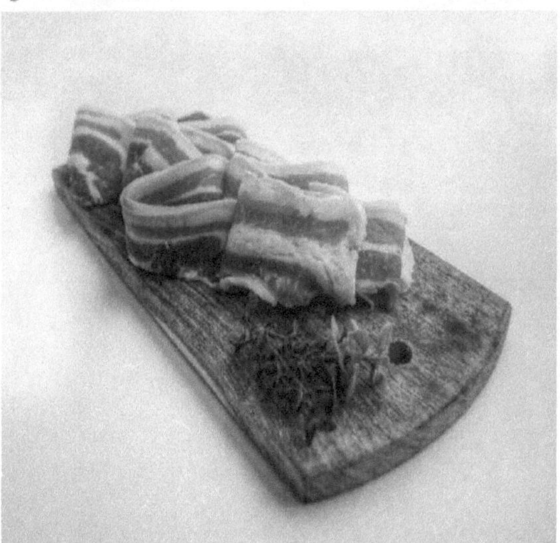

It's in the description: low-carb, high-fat diet. If it's in the definition, then that must mean as long as you keep your carb intake very low, you should be able to eat as much fat as you want, right? Well, as long as they are the "good" fats then definitely, the answer would be yes. In a Keto diet, unsaturated fats or the good fats are strongly recommended over saturated fats or bad fats. Some of the fats that are considered healthy come from: nuts, peanut butter, vegetable oil, avocado, and salmon.

It's alright if you're on and off Keto because you can still maintain the weight loss

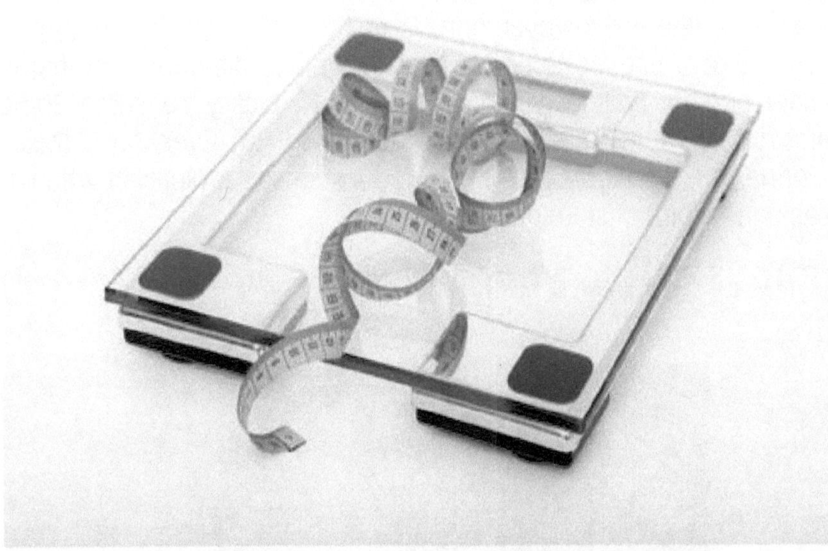

As is in the case of most fads, Keto is often misunderstood by most people. And because it *is* such a fad, people just jump into it without properly understanding the amount of dedication you have to put into actually making this diet work. For instance, people that are looking to lose weight often follow the Keto diet one day then eat carbs the next and still expect to keep the weight off. In reality, inconsistency with Keto will just cause you to gain all that weight back. Plus, by 'playing' at doing the Keto diet, you're not going to benefit from the effects of a sustained Ketosis. It goes without saying that if you plan to put yourself through a Keto diet, you have to stick with it to reap the rewards- otherwise, you're just depriving yourself of carbs for nothing. Consistency is key.

The amount of carbs everyone needs is the same

This aspect of diets is generally tricky. Diets tend to prioritize one macro (protein, carbs, fat) over the others in order to achieve a certain medical goal, and exactly how much of that macro needed to achieve the goal is different for everyone. With the keto diet, the amount of carbs you're supposed to consume may well be different from that of another person. Followers of the Keto diet typically consume 20-50 grams of carbohydrates a day, according to Everyday Health. Nevertheless, it's highly recommended to consult a dietician who will be able to tailor a custom diet plan for you.

Without carbs, your brain cannot function at all

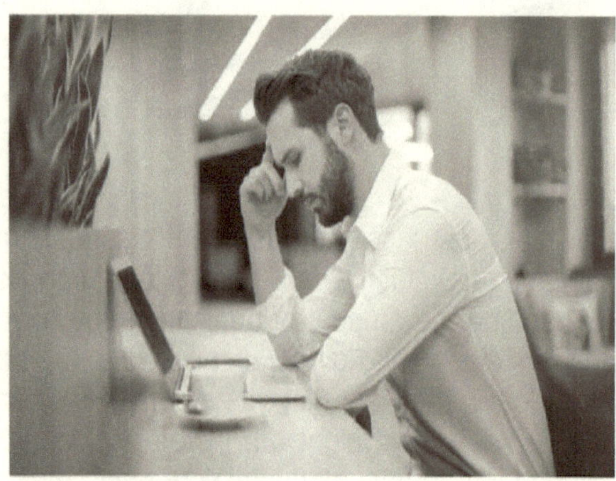

There is some truth to this notion. The people who believe this, claim that carbs are the preferred fuel for the brain and that it needs about 130 grams of it daily. And yes, there are really some cells in your brain that exclusively use carbs in the form of glucose as fuel.

 While that is true, there are also parts of your brain that can just use Ketones as fuel. If the Keto diet goes as intended, and carbs are reduced to an appropriate amount, Ketosis happens and a large part of your brain starts using Ketones for fuel instead of glucose. However, due to the fact that parts of your brain still need glucose, your body finds a workaround to address this demand. That wonderful brown organ called the liver comes to the rescue, and produces glucose out of protein and fat.

 So essentially, a large part of your brain can easily function on Ketones instead of glucose and the other parts that really need glucose can still get the same glucose without dietary carbs but with the aid of the liver. In fact, many people report having better brain function after adjusting to the low-carb diet.

Alcohol is off-limits when you're on Keto

Don't worry, you can still enjoy some wine or light beer when you're on Keto because alcohol isn't totally out of the question. Still, you should be a bit conscious of what kind of alcohol you drink and how much you drink. Although light beers and dry wine are fine because they have little to no carbs, they could still add up and therefore should be consumed in moderation. Additionally, your alcohol tolerance would likely be lower while on Keto, so it's definitely a good idea to watch how much you drink.

It hinders physical performance permanently and you won't be able to work out when on Keto

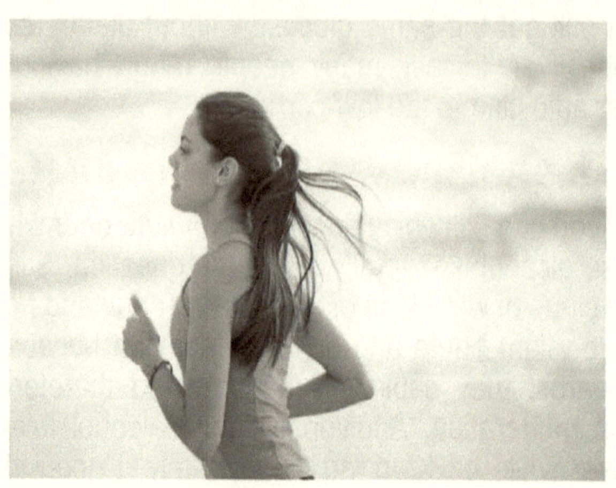

A lot of people believe that carbs are essential for physical performance and therefore indispensable in an athlete's diet. Although it's true that carbs are important for athletes, it's still possible for an athlete to perform at the same level on a low-carb diet. Because, the truth is that although reducing your carb intake does leave you feeling weaker in the beginning, the body always adapts, and this adjusting phase is usually only temporary. So it stands to reason that you will be able to work out the same way you did before being on Keto.

 But it's worth noting that you won't be feeling so great in the first few days or weeks, therefore it's best to stick to moderate exercise until your body adapts to the diet. With that being said, exercise greatly complements the Keto diet. Coupling Keto with exercise leads to significantly faster and more fat burn (around 2-3 times more), as well as good maintenance of blood glucose, and less fatigue in the long run.

Ketoacidosis and Ketosis are interchangeable terms

They might sound somewhat similar but there's a clear distinction between the two terms.

Ketosis is a metabolic process in which the body uses fat as energy instead of carbohydrates. Additionally, Ketosis is also a state in which mild amounts of Ketones are present. The keyword here is mild. In sharp contrast to this, Ketoacidosis is a complication of unmanaged type 1 Diabetes and it is a dangerous, potentially fatal condition.

According to Healthline, Ketoacidosis is a "condition resulting from dangerously high levels of ketones and blood sugar." This surplus in Ketones- around ten times the amount of when the body is in Ketosis- results in the blood becoming abnormally acidic and this, in turn, affects organ function.

In a nutshell, Ketoacidosis is a dangerous complication of a disease when your bloodstream gets flooded with immense amounts of Ketones; while Ketosis is a healthy metabolic state caused by a low-carb diet like the Keto diet.

The Keto diet is dangerous

Speaking of danger, many seem to dismiss the Ketogenic diet as a dangerous fad. In reality, the Ketogenic diet is not inherently dangerous and as long as you're careful, there's absolutely nothing to be concerned about.

It is, however, worth noting that it can technically be dangerous if one is not careful. According to Everyday Health, some of the potential downsides include: kidney stones, vitamin and mineral deficiencies, decreased bone mineral density, gastrointestinal distress, and an increased risk of higher cholesterol and heart disease.

Be careful to avoid these unwanted dangers by gradually easing into the diet, ensuring you stay hydrated, and hitting your daily macros. It does have downsides, but many beneficial things contain potential downsides. It's just a matter of actually understanding how it works and being cautious. Avoid rushing into it blindly, hoping that it is a magic weight loss formula. As with any diet, you should always be aware of its effects on your body, and consult your physician if you are concerned.

The Keto diet is the best way to lose weight

With all the hype surrounding the Keto diet, you can be forgiven for thinking it is the best way to lose weight. You may even think it is the only way to lose weight, sort of like the be-all, end-all of diets. Well, it definitely isn't the panacea of weight loss diets because it's different for everybody. In fact, a 2015 study published in the journal *Cell* posits that the blood sugar responses to the same foods vary among people so there is no diet that's perfect for everybody. Having said all that, the best diet is still the one you can consistently stick with.

Key Takeaways

The Keto diet has been shown to be very effective for losing weight and offers a lot of health benefits. Still, not everybody can benefit from Keto and misconceptions about it are common. Above all, it's always best to consult a doctor before trying out new diets.

Chapter 4

Step-by-Step Guide on Achieving Ketosis,

In this section, we will talk about how you can start your keto diet journey correctly. Please note that the steps outlined below are formulated with the general public in mind. If you have a pre-existing condition, then it's better for you to consult a health care provider before attempting the Ketogenic diet.

Step 1 – Determine Your Big WHY

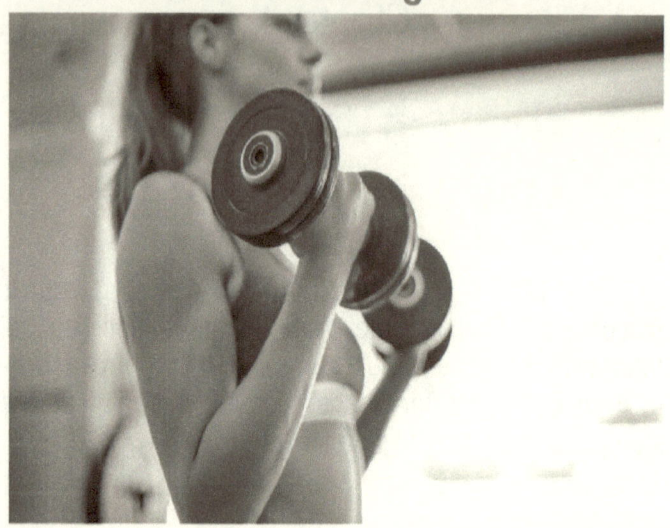

Determining your big WHY is the first step in any diet regimen – not just the keto diet. Ask yourself- why would I choose to deviate from my normal, and perhaps more satisfying diet? What do I want to achieve?

A person who wishes to change his or her diet typically wants to achieve one of the four goals:

- Lose weight
- Gain weight or build muscles
- Improve overall health
- Improve performance (for athletes)

You may be choosing the keto diet for the same reason as the majority: you want to lose weight. The good news is, not only will it help you to achieve this goal, but it can also bring about an improvement in overall health as well as an improved physical performance.

However, that said, if you want to build muscles, keto may not be the best option for you. This is because initially , carbohydrates have a huge role when it comes to muscle recovery. That's not to say you can't see results with keto, though. It's just that it may not seem that way to begin with. Once you have determined your big WHY, hold on to that thought as you progress along the diet's rocky road. As you may have already heard, the Ketogenic diet is NOT easy. A lot of people wind up giving up in the middle simply because it's too hard for them to follow the restriction in carbohydrates and the kinds of fats allowed.

As most inspirational speakers say: 'when you're about to give up, think about why you started'. So, take some time to deliberate about your goal, as it's really important.

Step 2 – Determine Your Total Caloric Goal

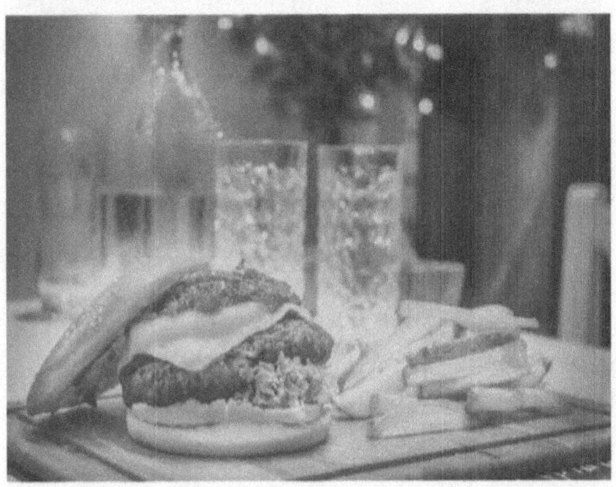

The next step after finding t your goal, is to calculate how many calories you need daily. The number of calories you need is definitely determined by your goal. For the purposes of this book, we're going to assume that you'd like to lose weight.

So how do you compute your caloric requirement if you want to lose weight? We'll cover that in this section, but first we need to discuss the calories themselves.

What Are Calories?

In this book, we mentioned the word "calories" in the first chapter when we said that "you have 3 main sources of calories – carbohydrates, fats, and proteins." But what exactly are calories and why are they so important for a person who would like to lose weight?

One definition of calories is this: it is the amount of energy needed to raise the temperature of 1 kg of water by 1 degree Celsius. That's quite complicated, right? So, we'll settle for this definition: calorie is energy. Without calories, we would not be able to survive.

Since calories are energy, we need to "burn" them to get energized. Think about climbing a mountain without proper sustenance – do you think you'd have enough energy to reach the summit? Probably not, if you didn't have enough calories to burn in the first place..

Calories are so crucial to our lives, that our body chooses to store them within muscle and fat tissues. If we eat food and we didn't use the calories in that food, then our body will "store them for future use." Where will our body store them? Most likely in those 'cushiony' places like the tummy, breast, buttocks, thighs, and even arms. Yup – unused calories or those calories that we didn't burn are stored as the unwanted fats or – the preferred option- the wanted muscles for those who want to beef-up.

It's a little morbid, but try imagining a person who has stopped eating for a really, really long time. You would probably see him as someone who's "still alive but is all skin and bones." Well, that imaginary person is "skin and bones" because, as he wasn't eating, the body naturally took his calorie reserves from his muscles and fats. It's the body's own way of making sure that we survive in case some circumstances prevent our intake of food.

Calories and Losing Weight

Now that we've cleared up the role of calories in survival, it'll be easier for us to understand their role in losing weight. In the Ketogenic diet, or in any other diet regimen, you need to work around your calories in order to maintain, gain, or lose weight.

Simply put, if you want to maintain weight, then you need to take in as many calories as you burn. If you want to gain weight, then you need to take in more calories than you burn. And finally, if you want to lose weight, you need to burn more calories than you take in.

Let's say that again: if you want to lose weight, then you need to burn more calories than you take in. That's the simplest formula, and it applies even in the Ketogenic diet.

Now, we've arrive to the most-awaited part:

How do we compute the amount of calories that we need?

Computing Your Total Caloric Goal

Before we teach you how to find your total caloric goal, we need to emphasize something – there's no one-size-fits-all formula for this. Your friend's caloric requirement is different from yours because you have different activities.

To compute your caloric goal, we need to take into consideration your activities because that's how we're going to find out how many calories you burn in a day. The term for the amount of calories we burn in a day is "total daily energy expenditure" or simply, TDEE.

Now, TDEE is broken down into several components, namely BMR, TEF, NEAT, and TEA. We will discuss all except for TEF, since you won't be able to use it to compute for the TDEE. TEF stands for Thermic Effect of Food or the calories we burn after digesting food.

BMR or Basal Metabolic Rate

The basal metabolic rate is the number of calories needed for the activities within our body. You see, you just don't need calories for when you move, bike, or hike. You also need calories for your heart to beat, for your lungs to perform gas exchange, or for your body to regulate temperature.

In other words, BMR is the amount of calories you need outside the calories you require to move.

NEAT or the Non-Exercise Activity Thermogenesis

NEAT is the number of calories you need if you want to make little movements, such as fidgeting, blinking, and moving your fingers.

TEA or Thermogenic Effect of Activity

TEA is the number of calories you need for more physically-taxing activities, such as running, jogging, or swimming.

Now, to compute your TDEE or the total amount of calories you need to consume in a day, you must multiply your BMR with your Activity Factor or AF. Here's a table for your AF:

Activity Level	Description	AF
Sedentary	Little to no exercise at all	1.1

Light	Light exercise 1 to 3 times weekly	1.2
Moderate	Moderate exercise 2 or more days weekly	1.35
Very Active	Hard exercise 3 or more days weekly	1.4
Extreme	Exercising twice a day or more	1.6

As for calculating your BMR, it's going to be a tedious process, so you can head over to this website for faster results: https://www.bodybuilding.com/fun/bmr_calculator.htm

Sample Computation:

Let's have an imaginary person who wants to lose weight as an example. Let's call her Jenny. Jenny has the following AF and BMR:

$$AF = 1.35$$

$$BMR = 1,451 \text{ calories}$$

Again, to get her TDEE (Total Daily Energy Expenditure), you need to multiply her AF with her BMR. In this example, her BMR is already provided. The computation goes like:

$$TDEE = 1.35 \times 1,451 \text{ calories}$$

$$TDEE = \underline{\textbf{1,958.55 calories}}$$

Take note that TDEE is her required caloric intake in a day – it's not her supposed caloric intake if she wants to lose weight. If Jenny would like to lose weight, then she needs to consume less than her TDEE.

Caloric Intake if you want to Lose Weight

Remember that if you want to lose weight, you need to consume fewer calories than your TDEE! But don't go around not eating because that's going to cost you a lot. Experts say cutting down your TDEE by 15 or 20 per cent is a good starting point. We call this "lessening down of TDEE" as a calorie deficit.

If you want a sustainable weight loss, or a weight loss that you can follow-through in the long run, then cut down your TDEE by 15% for at least 3 weeks and see how it goes. Simply use this formula:

$$TDEE \times 0.85$$

In Jenny's case, you can compute:

$$1{,}958.55 \times 0.85 = \underline{\mathbf{1{,}665.02}}$$

This means that for Jenny to lose weight, she needs to take **1,665.02** calories instead of her TDEE which is 1,958.55. She'd like to try this caloric goal for a period of 3 weeks to see if it's working or not. If it's working, she may go on with the same calorie level, or if she wants to see more results, she may cut down more of her calories (from 15%, she may now reduce it by 20%)

But the most crucial thing here is you must choose a calorie deficit that you are comfortable with. If you don't feel well when cutting your intake by 15%, try to cut it down by 10%. What's important is you're starting somewhere.

Step 3 – Incorporate Your Caloric Goal with the Ketogenic Diet

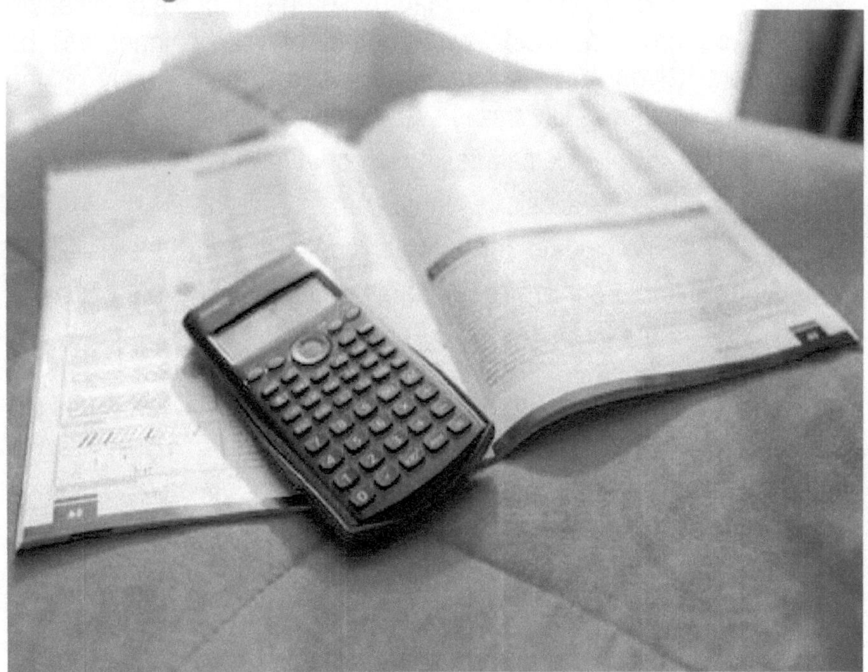

Phew! That was such a lengthy discussion, but hopefully, you got something good from it. To recap: remember that our first step is to identify your overall goal, and the second is to calculate your caloric goal.

The third step involves incorporating that caloric goal into the Ketogenic diet. And to do that, you need to think about your macros, or the sources of your calories; namely carbohydrates, fats, and proteins.

You see, your macros give different amounts of calories. Refer to the table below:

Macros	Calories
1 gram of carbohydrates	4
1 gram of proteins	4
1 gram of fats	9

Now, you need to identify which macros you need for Keto. What we mean is you have to decide where most of your calories will be coming from. Given that it's Keto, you'll need to heavily rely on fat; hence a ratio that looks like this is a good starting point:

60 – 75% calories must come from fat

15 to 30 % calories must come from protein

5 – 10% calories must come from carbohydrates

So, let's go back to our previous example, Jenny. Say Jenny wanted to start Keto and she wants *ease* her way into to. This means she doesn't want anything drastic, like getting 75% of her calories from fat, 20% from protein, and 5% from carbs. She feels that too few carbs will make her extremely weak and sick.

Again, she wants ease slowly into the diet regimen. So, Jenny decides to go for these macros:

60% of her calories will come from fats

30% of her calories will come from proteins; and

10% of her calories will come from carbohydrates

Now remember, her caloric goal is dictated by her goal to lose weight. It was: **1,665.02.** That means:

60% of 1,665.02 calories will come from fats

30% of 1,665.02 calories will come from proteins; and

10% of 1,665.02 calories will come from carbohydrates

The result would look like this:

999 calories will come from fats

500 calories will come from proteins; and

167 calories will come from carbohydrates

The only thing left to do now is to convert these figures into grams. You can use the table of Macros and Calories above. Simply divide 999, 500, and 167 by 9, 4, and 4 respectively. Here's the computation:

Fats: 999 calories / 9 calories = 111 grams of fats

Proteins: 500 calories / 4 calories = 125 grams of proteins

Carbohydrates: 167 calories / 4 calories = 41.75 grams of carbs

IMPORTANT: This computation only serves as an example. Some computations on the internet make use of your Body Mass Index and that could be even more accurate. Some even ask you to choose how many carbs you'd like to eat in a day, although many experts say that limiting it to 35 grams daily is okay! If in doubt, consult a doctor or a dietician.

Step 4 – Prepare Your Keto Checklist and Meal Plans

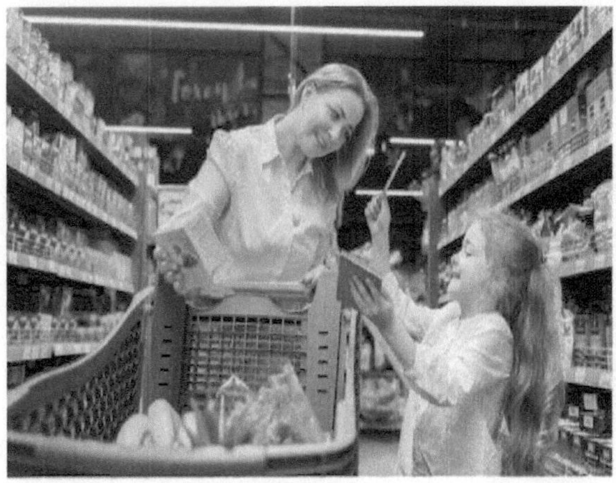

Since you have already established your goals, it's now time to prepare your Keto food checklists and meal plan. To do this, you'll need to know what foods are allowed in Keto and what foods aren't.

There will be no lengthy discussion for this section, since we will have separate chapters for the foods to eat and the foods to avoid. Additionally, we'll also have bonus recipes in this book. So watch out for that!

Step 5 – Prepare for Keto Flu

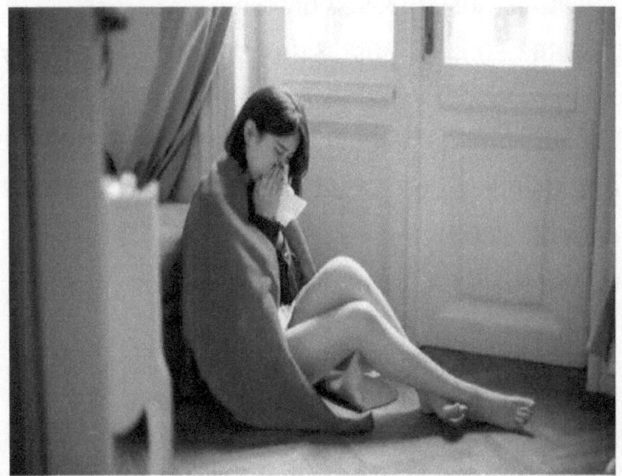

Once you have started the Ketogenic diet, remember that some changes in your body will happen. Don't be surprised!

Think about it: you are shifting from taking most of your calories from carbs to cutting carbs back to as little as 35 grams a day! In the first few weeks, you might feel really sick because of Keto.

This sickness is often called the Keto flu because of a variety of flu-like symptoms you experience as your body transitions from carb-burning to fat-burning. The symptoms include:

- Insomnia
- Sugar cravings
- Sore muscles
- Dizziness
- Confusion
- Irritability
- Nausea
- Cramping
- Stomach aches

Don't worry though. There are ways to feel better when you develop Keto flu. You can try to:

- Increase your water intake, and add a pinch of unrefined salt to one or two of those glasses of water.
- Increase the sodium, potassium, and magnesium levels in your diet.
- Turn to MCT(medium-chain triglyceride) oil for more energy
- Go for a morning walk, or other low-intensity exercise
- Get enough sleep
- Reduce stress through meditation

Finally, if you experience Keto flu DO NOT perform strenuous exercises and do not consume too much protein. You can also try to prevent Keto flu by gradually reducing your carb intake before you fully embrace the Ketogenic diet. What this means is: before officially starting on Keto, you can try reducing your carb intake until you reach your actual keto computations for fats, proteins, and carbs.

Key Takeaways

To start Keto:

Step 1 – Identify your goal or reason for going Keto.

Step 2 – Calculate your caloric goal; you can refer to the suggested website for easier computation.

Step 3 – Incorporate your caloric goal into the macros of the Ketogenic diet. You can refer to the recommended websites for easier calculations.

Step 4 – Prepare your Keto checklist and meal plans

Step 5 – Prepare for Keto flu

Remember that there's no one-size-fits-all formula for Keto. You need to consider YOURSELF when thinking about starting this diet regimen.

Chapter 5

Caution! Ketogenic Diet is Not For Everyone!

At this point, we have already discussed a lot of things about the Ketogenic diet. Based on this, you will now be aware of the incredible benefits that this new weight loss plan has to offer, which include:

- Weight loss of between 30 to 50 pounds or more can be achieved
- More energy to do the things that you love; and
- An improved blood sugar level

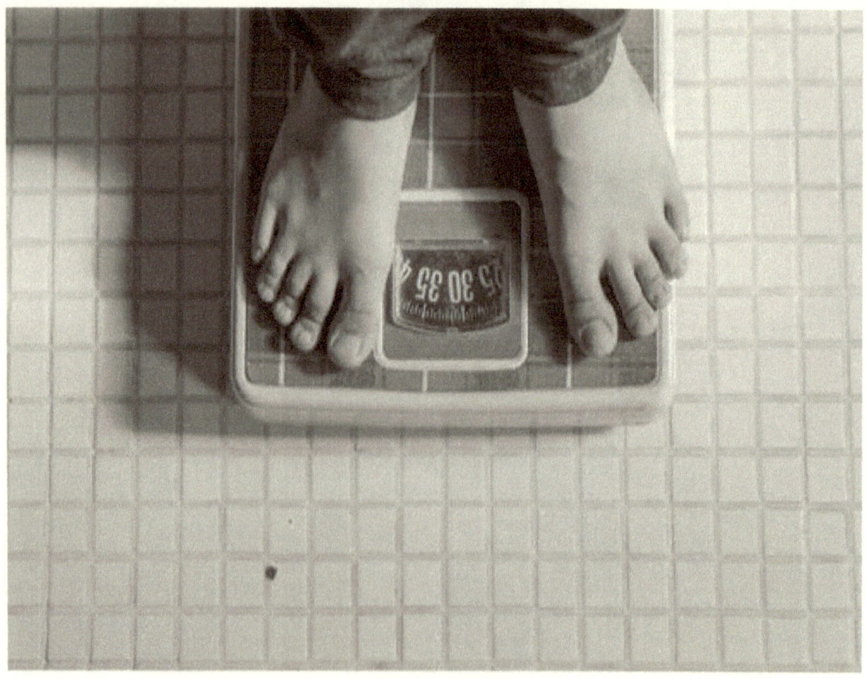

The thing is, despite its many benefits, the Ketogenic diet is NOT for everyone. If you are considering or even convincing yourself to do this diet, note that there are some instructions or directions which must be strictly followed. The strictness of the diet can make Keto seem too daunting or overwhelming for many people, but it is necessary if you are going to reap the rewards.

While you are using Keto, you need to:

- Check your blood sugar and ketone levels twice per day.
- Count the gram intake of protein every day.
- Check the percentage of calories you get from fat in comparison to those you get from other foods

In addition to these initially-taxing activities, you may also experience negative feelings like frustration and disappointment. If you had massive expectations of how Keto would work for you, and it hasn't worked as well as for as it may have done for others, then you may feel frustrated and disappointed. The frustration could be even greater if you know that you've tried your best to do it 'right'.

And at some point, you may question yourself about it and say "what have I done wrong?" There may even be this feeling of failure if you were not able to adhere to the diet perfectly.

You need to understand that you have not done anything wrong and you should feel broken or bad about this. The Ketogenic diet, as we have stated several times already, is not a one size meal plan that's good for everyone.

As Hippocrates said around 2600 years ago: 'one man's food is another man's poison' a fact which still holds true today. Any beginner who decides to go onto this diet must also recognize that each and every one of us is genetically different.

We all have a different DNA make up. We also live in different areas with differing climates and environments. We all have differing levels of stress to cope with on a daily basis. In addition, some of us have health issues and challenges to deal with too.. All these factors, and more, should be considered when we decide to go onto the Ketogenic diet.

According to Amy Gorin, a Registered Dietitian, although the Ketogenic Diet may seem to be the "trend" diet nowadays, we must also consider its adverse health effects. In her article entitled "The 11 Biggest Keto Diet Dangers You Need to Know", published on November 2, 2018, she shared the following risks:

- Muscle Loss or soreness
- Kidney Stones or kidney damage
- Occurrence of having Low Blood Sugar that can make it risky for people with diabetes
- As the Keto Diet is hard to follow, it can Lead to 'Yoyo' Dieting
- Dehydration and loss of electrolytes
- Nutrition deficiencies
- Bowel problems such as constipation
- Bad Breath
- Monthly periods may become irregular or completely stop under the Keto diet
- Lose sodium and electrolytes due to reduction in insulin
- High cholesterol and increased risk for heart diseases

With all these risk factors to consider, it is highly recommended that a doctor, health professional or expert be included as part of your plan if you are seriously considering the Ketogenic Diet. They will be able to provide guidance on your weight loss goal as well as advice on the right food for you, diet supplements you may need, and a personal maintenance program; as well as informing you of the specific effects that the keto diet may potentially have on your body..

They will also play a vital role in your meeting that optimum level of success in your weight goals and be there to guide you every step of the way. Their wisdom will prove invaluable if you intend to lose weight of more than 15 to 20 pounds, you have any health problems, or if you are on medication, since they can provide the necessary precautions and reminders. Without their assistance or at very least your own careful monitoring, the fat element of the keto diet, in particular, could prove to be disastrous.

As the popularity of the Keto diet has grown, there have been claims that it may not be the best long-term health plan. This is especially true for those who have a medical condition affected by fat intake, as the eating habits it promotes might lead mostly to heart problems.

How to know if Keto is for you:

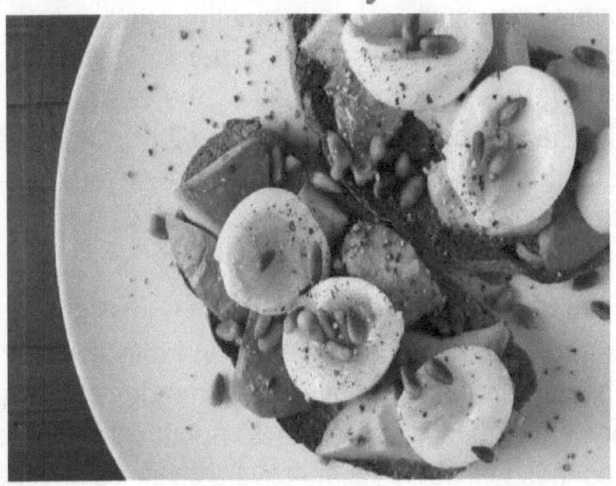

1. **Low-fat diets aren't working for you because you love high-fat foods**

   What if you just can't help yourself to that pork chop? Low-fat diets have been the go-to for many years, and are probably the most well-known of all diets. They can be effective too, but we have to admit- some of the tastiest foods are foods rich in fat and not everyone is willing to part with them.

   Enter the Keto diet. Low-carb and high-fat, this is rather like having your cake and eating it too. Why does this work? You see, your body has gotten used to using glucose from carbs for fuel. What the Keto diet essentially does is force the body to burn fats instead of carbs. This is achieved by drastically reducing your carb intake while increasing the fats, hence the low-carb and high fat diet. But it's important to note that the Keto diet highly encourages healthy fats like avocados, whole eggs, nuts, fatty fish, and yogurt, to name a few. So if for some reason you can't shed those extra pounds with low-fat diets, the Keto Diet might be the diet for you.

2. If you're experiencing inflammation

Low-carb diets like Keto are far less inflammatory than diets rich in sugar. Not only does a diet high in refined sugar cause obesity, but studies show that it also causes low-grade inflammation. It contributes so much to inflammation that simply removing carbohydrates, refined sugar, and gluten from your diet is enough to lower the inflammation present in the body. Fortunately, the Keto diet has no need for sugar in its diet because ketosis uses fats instead of sugar for energy. Therefore, if you cut out sugar or glucose from your diet and replace it with Keto food, you'll have fewer aches and pains..

3. If you need a quick and effective way to lose weight

If done properly, Keto can be a fast and effective way to lose up to 10 pounds in just a month. The average rate of safe weight loss for Keto dieters is about 4 to 10 pounds per month or around 1 to 2 pounds per week. As effective as it is, it's important to keep in mind that it only works as a short-term solution.

According to *Mission Lean* co-founder Lyuda Bouzinova, if keeping the weight off in the long run doesn't concern you, the Keto diet can work as a short-term solution for losing weight quickly. She further states that once you start to gain weight again after Keto, you should try a more sustainable weight loss method.

4. If you're insulin-resistant

When the cells in your fat, muscles, and liver lack the ability to properly respond to insulin because you have insulin resistance, they won't be able to use glucose for fuel. To compensate, the pancreas produces more insulin. Eventually, your blood sugar will be elevated to dangerously high levels and this puts you at a huge risk for type 2 diabetes and other health problems.

The Keto diet may be able to increase your insulin sensitivity, according to a 2005 study led by Guenther Boden. The study found that they were able to drastically increase insulin sensitivity (by 75%) in 10 subjects with insulin resistance. So if you're insulin resistant, the Keto diet might increase your insulin sensitivity at least for the short-term.

5. **If you can actually commit to the diet**

Simply put, the best way to reap the rewards of the Keto diet is to be consistent. The more consistent you are, the better the results will be. One of the most common misconceptions about the Keto diet is that it's okay to seesaw on Keto. This isn't true because when you adhere to the Keto diet rules one day then eat carbs the next, it will just lead to weight gain, thereby invalidating your efforts. At the end of the day, no matter how much evidence there is to suggest that Keto is good for you, but you aren't diligent enough, it's simply not going to work. Remember - consistency is the key to success.

How to know if Keto is not for you:

1. **Your doctor or dietician advised against it**

    As the risks of Keto vary from person to person, it would be wise to consult your doctor. And while a lot of doctors would recommend Keto to treat some health conditions, they are also aware that some people just shouldn't go on it.

    For instance, Fiber helps fight digestive problems so if you have a personal history of digestive issues like an ulcer or colon cancer, doctors would recommend that you would be better off without Keto because Keto doesn't allow foods rich in Fiber. Fiber is important for indigestion and constipation, according to the National Institutes of Health, so Keto is simply a health risk in this situation.

2. **You don't enjoy food anymore when you're on Keto**

    Do you find yourself loathing mealtimes? Does eating feel more like a chore you have to get over with so you can get on with your day? If you said yes to those questions when you're on Keto, then that's a huge problem, especially when you describe yourself as a "foodie".

    Food is part of human culture and it is meant to be enjoyed. We don't eat just to survive anymore. We also eat because it tastes good and makes us feel good. You're supposed to eat what you enjoy, albeit in moderation. For most people, dietary preference is a factor when deciding what diet you want to be on because you're far more likely to stick with it and therefore, be successful with it if you're happy to eat the foods the diet recommends.

According to Registered Diet Nutritionist Megan Ware, you shouldn't try to go against what your body wants because although you may be able to eat that way but in time, you'll feel restricted.

3. You go on cheat days when on the diet

This is a consequence of not enjoying food anymore when you're on the diet. You stray from the diet when you feel overly restricted or if you don't like the food you're supposed to eat. When a cheat day becomes necessary, it's only another reason that Keto isn't right for you.

Consistency is key when it comes to the Keto diet and cheat days disrupt your consistency leading to an on and off scenario.. Not only is being on and off the diet just a waste of time, but it could also have adverse effects on your health..

A 2019 study published in the health journal *Nutrients* indicates that Keto diet cycling can cause damage to blood vessels. On top of that, not being able to decide how you want to live your own life is not a healthy mentality. If you find yourself restarting your diet every week, you're not doing it right and it's obviously not the right thing for you..

4. You acquire issues with your period when you started the diet

Evidence shows that it is possible for the Keto diet to affect hormone signaling in women. It can wreak havoc on your hormones, thus causing you to miss your period for several months. If you are not menstruating and not pregnant, this is a sign that the Keto diet is too restrictive for your body type and is not for you.

5. You're not fine with social isolation

When you're out eating with friends, do you feel left out because you're restricted from eating whatever they are all eating? Or maybe you find yourself hesitating to even go to family gatherings because you know you're just going to say no to that sweet apple pie your grandma serves. Either way, it's quite possible for you to feel socially isolated because of your restrictive diet. Culturally and socially, food plays an important role, as it brings you and your loved ones closer together. If Keto gets in the way of your connecting with friends and family, it's a sign that you need to reconsider.

6. **You're not even losing weight while on the diet**

Your favorite celebrity made it seem so easy losing weight with Keto and your friend has been boasting about the weight they lost using Keto, but you just aren't losing anything at all. RDN Megan Ware says that people tend to feel guilty when they're on a diet yet still don't lose weight. She adds that diets set an arbitrary set of rules that are not primarily based on you, your lifestyle, your genetics, or diet preferences. It's the diet that's failing you, not the other way around. Fortunately, you can consult a registered dietician to help you make a custom weight loss diet that's tailored to your preferences, lifestyle, and genetics. This way, you have a better chance of reaching your weight loss goals. There's always hope.

7. **When you have conditions preventing you from metabolizing fatty acids**

People who suffer from congenital health conditions such as Porphyria and Pyruvate Carboxylase Deficiency should stay away from Keto. This is because Keto is a high-fat diet and people who have the aforementioned conditions are unable to metabolize fatty acids. So in a nutshell, if you have this condition, you cannot utilize fat as energy, which is the main goal of a Keto diet.

What to do when Keto isn't for you?

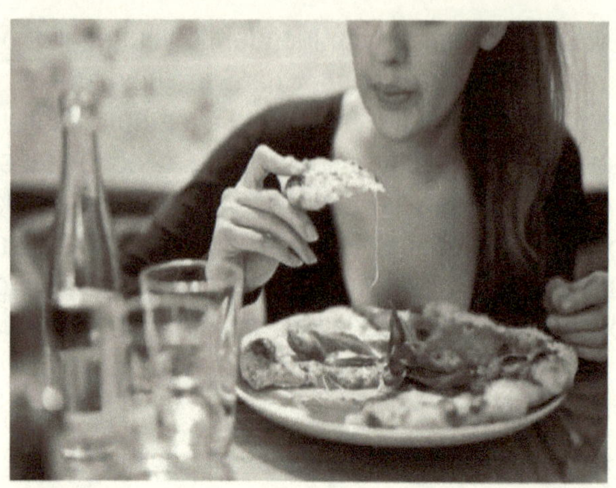

So you've read the list and unfortunately Keto is impractical or downright dangerous for you. The good news is there's still hope for you to lose weight. Believe it or not, there are numerous diets out there designed for different people with different needs. And even if somehow none of those popular diets are a fit for you, a registered nutritionist can always help you properly tweak those diets to create a custom made diet plan for you. So don't despair; your weight loss journey doesn't stop at Keto. Here is an alternative to consider:

The Mediterranean Diet - Widely regarded as one of the healthiest diets, this heart disease-preventing diet heavily emphasizes fruits, whole grains, vegetables, and legumes. It also encourages low-fat dairy products, poultry, and some vegetable oils while restricting highly processed foods, added sugars, refined carbs, and saturated fats. Not only will this diet steadily and gradually help you lose weight, but it also promotes healthy eating patterns that help stave off the nasty diseases linked to obesity.

Key Takeaways

Just because a lot of people are saying that Keto worked well for them, it doesn't mean that Keto is the one for you. Try to assess and re-assess yourself. Is Keto right for you? Can you endure the highly demanding activities that come with it? Don't be afraid to answer NO - you do still have other options. However, if you feel that the Keto diet is for you, great!

Chapter 6

Foods to Eat

Finally! We're in the chapter where you'll find the best foods to eat should you decide to try the Ketogenic diet. Think of this chapter as a detailed grocery shopping list. As we enumerate the foods that are great for Keto, we will also explain their value in a way which you may find useful in your journey to shed pounds.

PRO-TIP: Remember what we said earlier, about the Keto flu? That you can prevent having it by easing your way into the Keto diet? Well, you do that by gradually removing high carb foods *before* you start the keto approach. So, before we give you the grocery list – here's a challenge for you. A month or so before starting keto, remove the following from your fridge and pantry:

- Sodas or any drink that has sugar in it
- Cakes and other pastries
- Packaged snacks
- Super sweet treats

You don't need to get rid of them all at once. Let's say for week 1, you'll give away all your sodas. For week 2, you'll give away all your pastries to your neighbour. And the trend goes on until your pantry is left with empty space for all the good foods we're going to talk about in this chapter!

List of Foods to Eat to Achieve Ketosis

Seafood

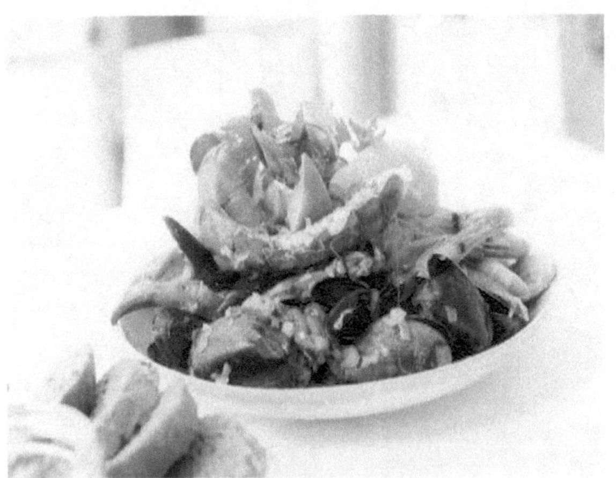

There are two reasons why seafood and fish are perfect if you want to start your Ketogenic diet journey: firstly, they are filled with a lot of vitamins and minerals that are important to keep you healthy, and secondly they are almost carb-free! Most seafood, like albacore, sardines, and mackerel, contain selenium, potassium, B vitamins, and guess what? Proteins!

If you're looking for good fats, that are protein-rich and almost carb-free, seafood is the way to go!

Here's the Top 10 list you can count on:

1. Clams
2. Tuna
3. Crabmeat
4. Squid
5. Sole
6. Shrimp
7. Herring
8. Lobster
9. Salmon
10. Mussels

Vegetables

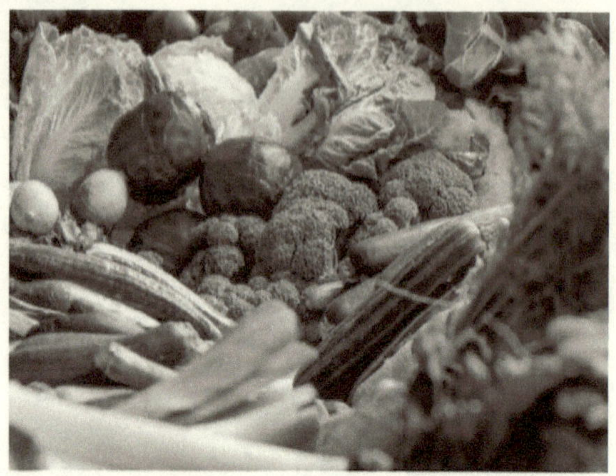

So, we all know that veggies are healthy! Leafy greens in particular, have a lot of things to boast about when it comes to nutrient content that boosts our immune system. However, when it comes to the Ketogenic diet, vegetables are quite tricky.

You see, some vegetables are high in carbs, and when you want to be in ketosis, you don't want that, right?

So, what we are looking for are non-starchy veggies that are low in carbs, but high in vitamins and minerals as well as antioxidants that can protect our cells from the dangers of free radicals.

Here are the Top 10 Low-Carb Veggies

1. Lettuce
2. Zucchini
3. Spinach
4. Kale
5. Cucumber
6. Celery
7. Cabbage
8. Cauliflower
9. Broccoli
10. Asparagus

Dairy Products

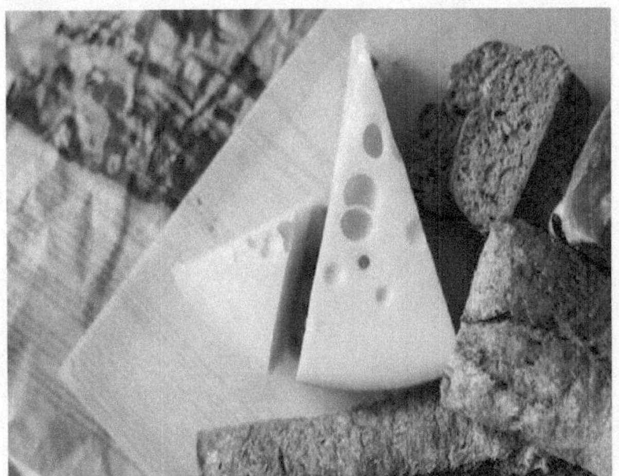

Dairy products, like cheese, often have very few carbohydrates in them. Additionally, they are high in fat, which is perfect for Keto. However, if you're suffering from any kind of disease that prompts you to avoid saturated fats, be careful with cheese. According to reports, just a slice of cheese can fill up about 40% of the daily requirement for saturated fats.

Another great thing about cheese and other dairy products is that they are rich in calcium, which is great for the bones and teeth.

Here are your Top 10 Cheese and Dairy Products

1. Cream cheese
2. Cheddar cheese
3. Cottage cheese
4. Greek yogurt
5. Goat's cheese
6. Feta
7. Parmesan
8. Mozzarella
9. Butter
10. Blue cheese

Aside from these dairy products and cheeses, we should also include milk and yogurt.

When choosing milk, consider high-fat or full-fat varieties. The same goes for cream: choose heavy or sour cream.

As for yogurt, go for the Greek kind. Greek yogurt is perfect, especially if you're looking for a great snack. What makes it even more perfect is that Greek yoghurt contains probiotics which are good for the digestive system. This is because probiotics add good, live bacteria to the body.

Fruits

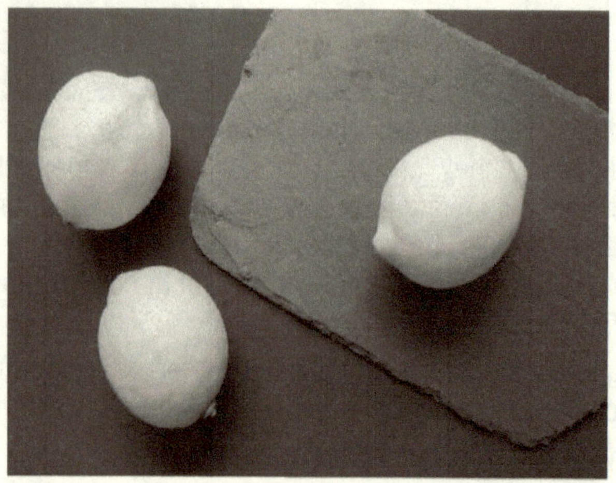

Now, you might be wondering, fruits are sweets, right, so am I allowed to eat fruits? The short answer is "No", most fruits are not okay for the Ketogenic diet. But a diet without fruits is quite sad not only because you'll be missing the colors and taste, but also because you'd be missing out on the nutrients they contain. So, is there a way around it?

The good news is, there is!

According to Everyday Health, you just need to choose the low-carb and, if possible, high fat ones! Here are the best 5 of fruits for the Ketogenic diet!

1. **Avocados.** Avocados are great if you want to achieve ketosis! They have low sugar content, but also contain about 12 grams of fat. The avocados' best asset, however, is its taste! It's versatile, too! You can include it in salads, smoothies, or even

desserts!

2. **Watermelon.** Some people feel that watermelons are only meant for summer, but they're actually an all-time favorite! Like avocado, they're also tasty and can be eaten on their own or as a part of a smoothie or in shake recipes. They're low in carbs but high in water – perfect if you want to keep your hydration up..

3. **Lemon.** And who can forget lemons? Lemons are famous for their health benefits- that's why people often use them as an ingredient in the home remedy for colds.. They are great for Keto too, because they are low in sugar but high in vitamin C and antioxidants! On top of everything else, lemons are also versatile in the sense that you can include them in meals, salads, and drinks!

4. **Strawberries**. Another great fruit you can eat in moderation are strawberries. To ensure that you're not eating too much, it's best to slice them and eat them together with a Keto-friendly dessert.

5. **Tomatoes**. Okay, so most people do not consider tomatoes as fruits, but technically, they are fruits! If you're not fond of eating them on their own, there are a lot of ways to eat tomatoes. From salads to sandwiches and as an integral part of meals, you name it! There are a lot of recipes that call for tomatoes!

Meat

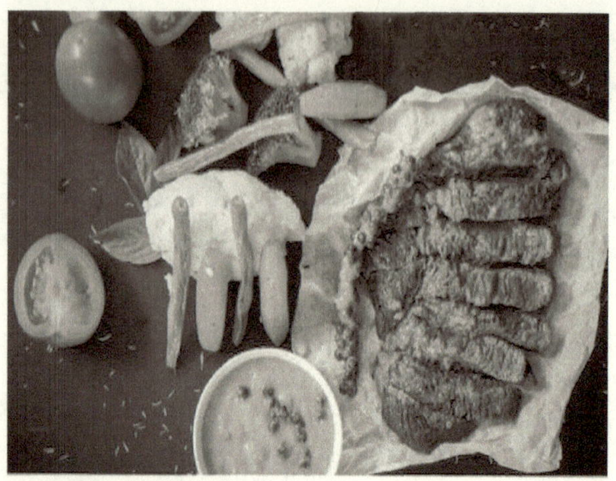

Okay, we can't talk about Keto without talking about meat and poultry. As you need to adhere to a low-carb and high fat diet, you are going to rely heavily on meat and poultry (aside from seafood, that is).

However, before we proceed with the list, please remember that you need healthy fats. That means less saturated and trans fat. As much as possible too, eat less of processed and preserved meats as they may be cured with sugars, which you don't want to add while you're on the Keto diet.

Here are the Top 5 Meats and Poultry for Keto:

1. Beef
2. Ham
3. Lamb
4. Pork
5. All Poultry

While we're on the topic of meat, let's also discuss EGGS. Almost all people who successfully accomplished ketosis have also relied heavily on eggs. That's because eggs are all-around food, you can have them for breakfast, lunch, dinner, and snacks. Eggs also have a lot of proteins, vitamins and minerals, as well as antioxidants.

If you're someone who is looking for a food that won't remind you that you're dieting, eggs are probably your best option.

Nuts and Seeds

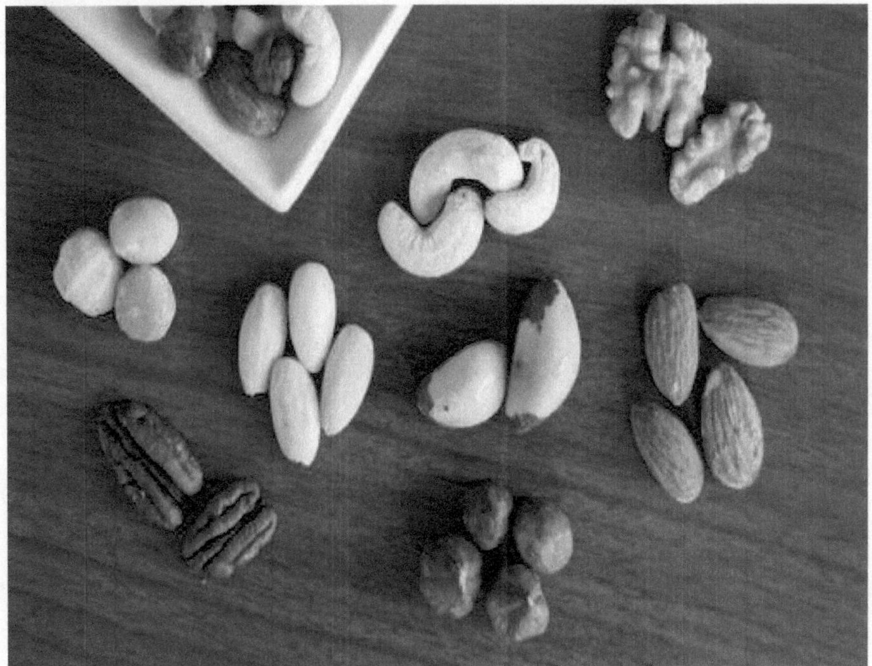

So here's the thing about nuts – they are great for peanut butter. But that's not all! High in protein, high in fats, and low in carbs: these characteristics make nuts and seeds perfect for the Ketogenic diet.

Just a little word of caution, though, if you're going to choose nuts and seeds, stay away from the ones with added sugar. Usually, the labels will read "sugar-coated" , so always read the labels!

Lastly, if you feel that nuts are boring, look at this Top 8 List. You'll see that you have a lot of choices:

1. Brazil nuts
2. Walnuts
3. Flax seeds
4. Sesame seeds
5. Sunflower seeds
6. Hazelnuts
7. Macadamia nuts

8. Pecans

Oils

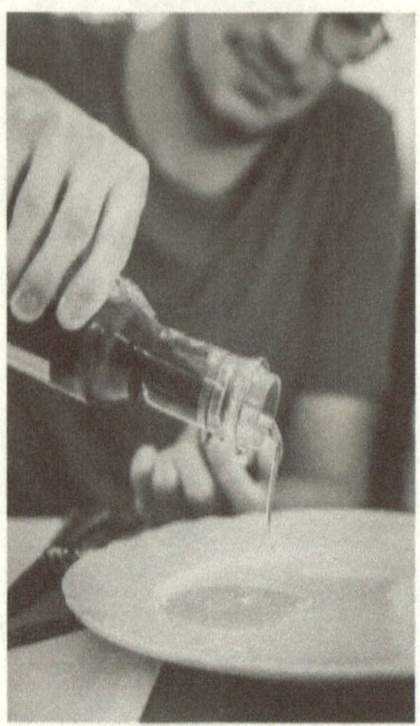

And finally, we're going to talk about fats and oils. Oils are important because they cook the food AND they add flavour. Here's a list of different oils and fats you can rely on:

1. MCT oil
2. Mayonnaise
3. Avocado oil
4. Coconut butter
5. Olive oil

Now that you have a list of the things that you can include in your grocery list, we will talk about the items you MUST NOT include in your shopping.

Key Takeaways

Whoever says that Keto is boring hasn't seen the variety of keto recipes. With all these food items, there's no reason why you cannot enjoy each mealtime. Aside from the recipes that we will be providing later, you also have the option to search online! Just keep this list close to you whenever you plan on grocery shopping.

Chapter 7

Foods to Avoid

I t's not enough that you know what you can eat, you also need to know about the foods you need to avoid:

Fruits

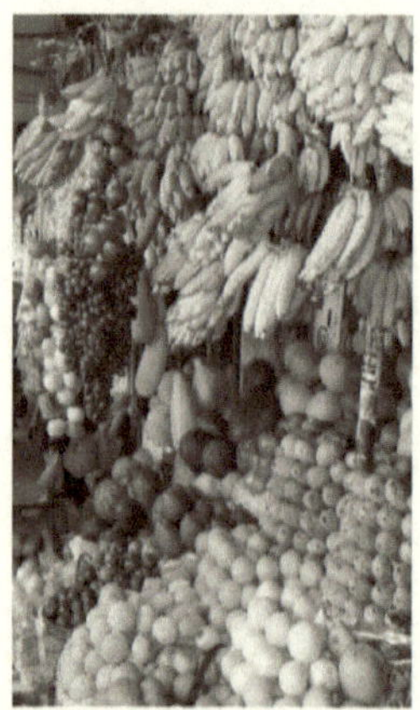

Remember when we discussed that there are only a handful of fruits you can eat? Well, that's because most fruits have sugars in them which are not great for Keto.

Sweet and starchy fruits like bananas, mangoes, apples and such, should be avoided.

Starches

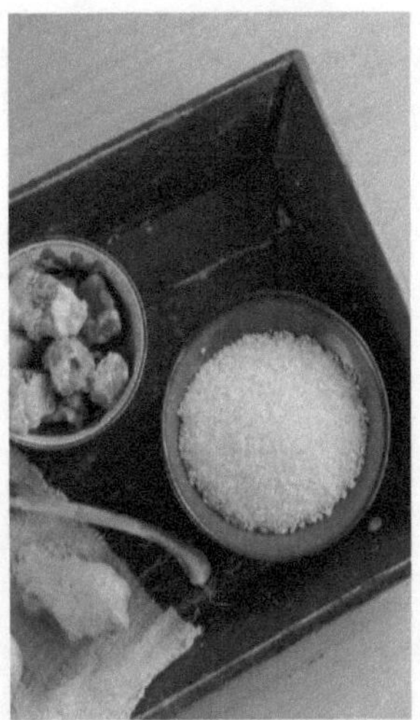

Grains are filled with carbs, so it's best to stay away from them whenever possible. If you're on the keto diet, most people would consider eating white rice and pasta to be a sin! However, because of technology, many products now are "Keto-safe" despite being considered as "rice or pasta."

 If you're keen on eating rice, pasta, or bread, be sure to check if they are Keto-safe first. Remember that most are filled with the dreaded, carb-rich starch!

Grains

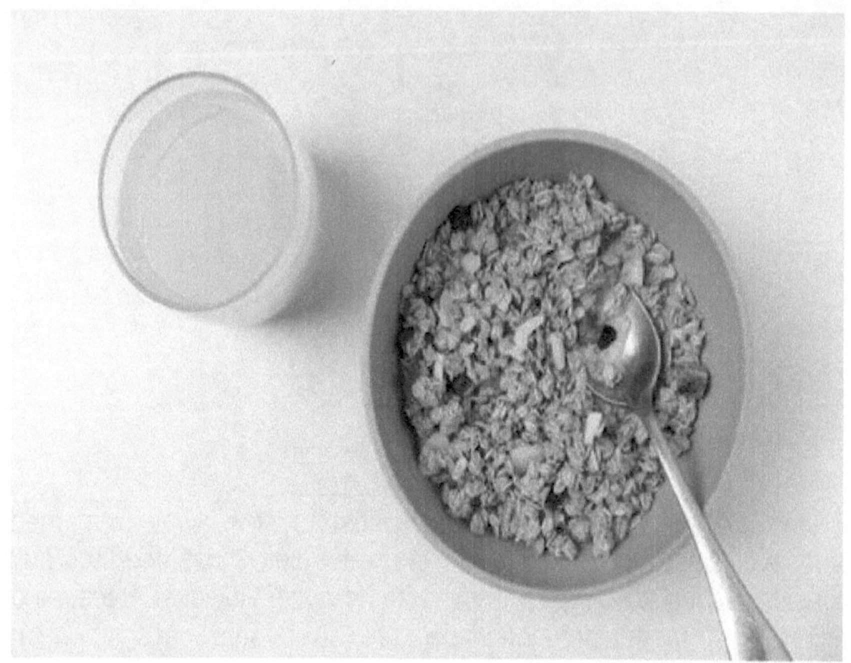

Some people who are switching to a healthier lifestyle tend to forego starches, but patronize grains such as rye, quinoa, barley, and buckwheat. However, if you're on the keto diet, you should avoid them as much as possible. They, too, are rich in carbs.

Sweets

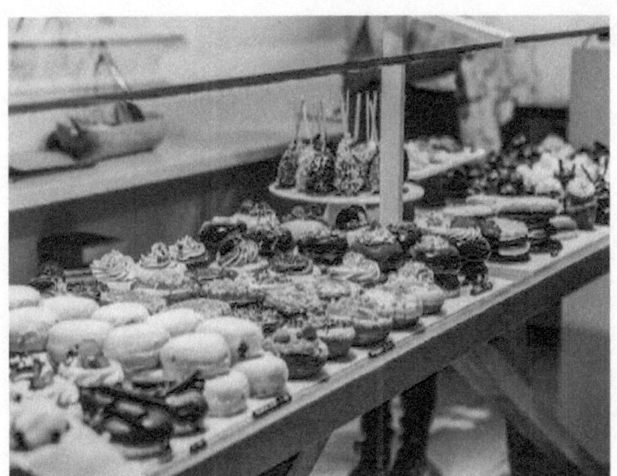

When you're on the keto diet, avoid anything sweet! That means chocolate, candies and pastries! However, nowadays, some companies and small businesses are selling Keto-friendly pastries. Find a trusted store that can cater for your sweet tooth.

 If you're worried, you can make your own pastries by using Keto friendly ingredients.

 Also, take note of sweeteners, such as honey, maple syrup, aspartame, and corn syrup. They are also a no-no for Keto.

 Finally, any foods (especially snacks) that have the word "sweetened" in them must be avoided.

Condiments

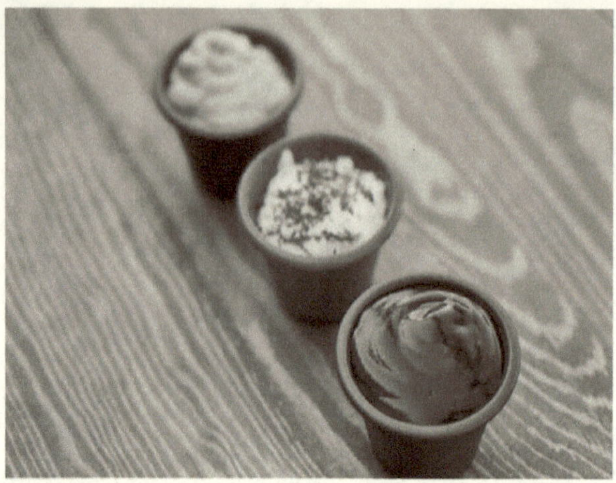

When we're on a diet, we don't often pay attention to condiments – after all, they're not "the main dish." They couldn't do anything to jeopardize our goal to lose weight.

Well, that's kind of wrong.

Condiments have calories, too, and when you add them haphazardly and without thought as to quality and measurement, they may prevent you from going into ketosis sooner.

On the Ketogenic diet, try to avoid condiments such as tomato sauce, barbecue sauce, ketchup, hot sauce, and some salad dressings that contain added sugar.

Additionally, some oils are also quite not acceptable. Please refrain from using canola, grapeseed, soybean, and sesame oil.

Key Takeaways

This is such a short list compared to the one that we discussed when talking about the foods you *can* include in keto diet. It's going to be hard at first, but in time, especially when you're already seeing the results, you'll find it's worth it.

Chapter 8

What about Drinks?

Here's a really sensitive topic – drinks.

Don't get us wrong, it's not like it's going to be a complicated topic; let's just say that it's a little touchy, because many people don't actually count what they drink.

And that's even more reason why being mindful of your drinks is important.

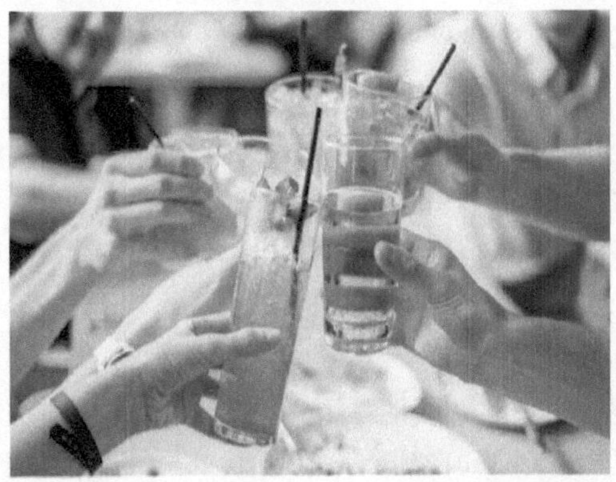

Just imagine this: you are very careful with your foods – you eat low-carb, high fat meals and snacks, you add more servings of non-starchy veggies and fruits, and then you binge on sugary drinks because you feel that they don't count.

They do. And the more you refuse to accept that they count a whole lot, the longer it'll take you to be in the state of ketosis.

Many doctors would like to point this out to you: don't drink your calories!

Best Drinks for the Ketogenic Diet

Drink More Water

Remember this: it doesn't matter what your diet is, water remains the best fluid for the well-being of your body. If you really want to get serious with Keto, experts suggest that you must always keep a bottle of plain water within reach.

Choose your Tea Wisely

When on the Ketogenic diet, can I drink tea? The short answer is *yes, you can*, the long answer is *yes, you can, but you need to be careful with your choice.*

Let's face it, not all people can stand drinking water and water alone. At some point, you'll really crave something with flavor. When it's cold, you'll most probably look for hot drinks, and tea is a healthy option.

Well, as long as the tea is low-carb and calorie-free. No worries, most teas pass these criteria, but just in case, check the labels.

Another great reminder is- refrain from adding anything like sugar or honey to your cup of tea!

Try Seltzer or Sparkling Water

If you're looking for a way to spice up your water, try seltzer and sparkling water. They are also calorie-free. However, be careful with tonic. Tonic looks clear and safe, but it actually has a lot of sugars in it.

Your Choices of Caffeine

Many people across all dietary regimens are dependent on coffee, especially in the morning, but is coffee okay when you're trying to achieve ketosis?

Experts say it is, AS LONG AS you take it straight and black.

While it's true that many can do that, bitter coffee is quite daunting for some.

The good news is- you can add a swirl of heavy cream. Remember don't add anything else other than heavy cream, and definitely not sugar, to your cup of morning coffee.

Milk

So, as we mentioned earlier, milks which are not full cream are a big no-no. But you also have another option – nut milk varieties.

The best options in this area, are coconut milk, almond milk, and cashew milk. They are all very low in carbs, as long as you choose the unsweetened variety. But as always, check the labels.

Another good thing about nut milks is that they are usually fortified with vitamins and minerals.

Missing Soda? Try Kombucha!

Alright, so let's face the truth: sodas are a big part of some people's lives. You drink them together with meals or when you're simply craving for something cold and sweet. The thing is- we know that sodas are packed full with sugars.

Definitely not a drink for someone who's on the keto diet.

If you're looking for an alternative, try Kombucha. It is a fermented tea that's also a good source of probiotics.

Take note that Kombucha is not completely devoid of carbs (in fact, many experts say that it contains quite a lot), however, it is still a better option when compared to sodas.

Even so, try not to drink kombucha on a regular basis if you can avoid it.

What about Alcohol?

This is one question Keto beginners are always curious about: what about alcohol? Can I still drink alcohol when I go out with friends after a long, hard day at work?

Well, guess what? You can take the occasional sips of wine as long as you include the alcohol calories in your daily count. And of course, you cannot party all night, every night!

Additionally, when it comes to alcohol, some types are preferable to others. For instance, vodka, gin, rum, and whiskey have 0 grams of carbohydrates per serving of 1 ounce.

No matter what you do, don't resort to beer, cocktails, and wine coolers.

Key Takeaways

Water is still the best drink if you want to lose weight using the Ketogenic diet. Sure, you can drink the other types mentioned above, but remember to do so in strict moderation.

 As much as possible, when you're counting your calories, especially your carbs, include your drinks in the computation.

Chapter 9

Practical Tips When It Comes to Ketogenic Diet

Now that you know about the step-by-step process, as well as which foods and drinks to eat and avoid, let's talk about some practical tips that you may find useful as a beginner.

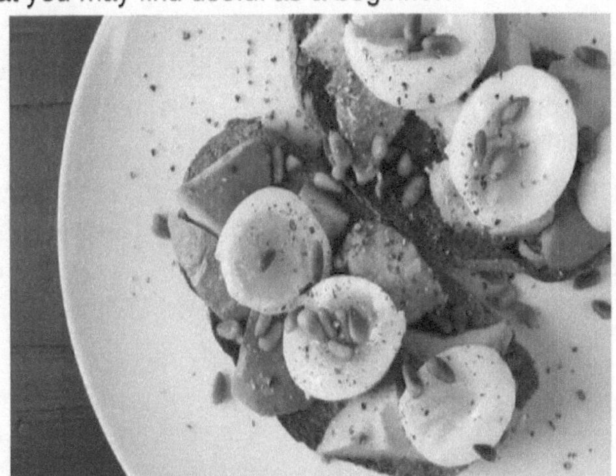

We will divide these practical tips into 3: the first will be practical tips to help you to reach ketosis, the second will be the tips to help you to identify when you're in ketosis, and the last will be to assist you with your long-term Keto plan.

How to Reach Ketosis?

When you're in ketosis, it means that your body is in that highly desirable fat-burning state. Sure, you can achieve ketosis by taking into considerations the guidelines we talked about earlier, but what other tips would you find useful?

Up the Ante in Your Physical Activities

The only way you're going to burn the calories you have in your excess fats is through physical activities. So, if you can, up the ante in your physical activities. There are a lot of ways to do this:

First, you can hit the gym. Typically, they'll have instructors there who you can talk to about your goals, and of course, how you are starting on the Ketogenic diet. This is important because they will know what to do about your physical performance and encourage you to stretch yourself. You'll have guidance about whether you're doing too much or too little.

Now, if you're not fond of gyms, you can also exercise from home. Surf the internet for instructional videos- there are plenty of them out there, but it's preferable to use workouts that people who are starting Keto are using.

Finally, don't forget that the little things matter. For instance, walking the short distance from the parking lot to the office, carrying a bag of groceries, and playing with your dog in the neighbourhood – these are all great activities to start with.

Just a quick, but important reminder: don't exercise when you're sick or not feeling well. And most definitely don't exercise when you're having chest pain or shortness of breath. If you experience these worrying symptoms, it's important to consult your physician.

Try to Add More Coconut Oil to Your Diet

Ask people who are no longer new to the Ketogenic diet, and they'll probably advise you to have MCT oil. MCT stands for medium-chain triglycerides. These are the kind of fats that are directly taken up by the liver and used immediately for energy. In other words, they are easily converted to ketones.

Guess what? Coconut oil contains MCT and is often more readily available.

However, if you want to, you can look for actual MCT oil in stores.

Try Fasting

Alright, I know it sounds excessive, since you're already on a low-carb diet, but it can help to try fasting for short periods. A lot of experts say that many people reach the state of ketosis in between meals, i.e. in the time when they are not eating anything.

However, more studies are needed to confirm this, so it's best to proceed with fasting with caution.

Don't Stray from the Basics

Finally, the most important tip in order to reach the state of ketosis is to follow the basics – that means having low-carb foods, healthy fats, and proteins.

And don't forget to have variety, as it will help to ensure that you remain healthy.

How to Know When You're in Ketosis?

Now, we've arrived at a very really interesting question – how do you know when you're in ketosis? Well, the easy thing to do is to test for ketones, right? In the absence of a testing kit, you can rely on the following signs and symptoms.

You're Losing Weight

The first sign is weight loss, and wouldn't that be a very welcome development? When you're in ketosis, you're in that state where your body is burning fat effectively. So that means you'll notice that you're indeed losing weight.

You Feel Thirsty

Another sign that you're in ketosis is you feel thirsty. This is probably because, initially, your body will be losing 'water weight'.

Although you might feel happy about feeling thirsty as it could mean that you're reaching ketosis, don't forget to drink plenty of water. Dehydration is a serious condition and it must not be taken lightly.

You Feel Unwell

Okay, so that definitely doesn't sound good, but the experts say that feeling unwell could be a sign of ketosis (Keto 'flu). The question is: what things are you going to feel?

Due to the depletion of electrolytes from dehydration, you would experience cramping and muscle spasms. . So, don't wait until you're dehydrated. If you feel thirsty, drink water.

You may also complain about having headaches. Experts say that most people experience headaches from day 1 to day 7 after switching to the Ketogenic diet. However, some people experience headaches for longer than 7 days.

One important point: if your headaches persist or become intolerable, consult your doctor. Remember that headaches could be a signs of many different conditions from migraines to hypertension or even an aneurysm.

During ketosis, you may also feel weak and tired. And that isn't really surprising, is it? After all, you're making a big change – from using carbohydrates to using fats. Carbohydrates, as we discussed earlier, are easier to digest and turn into energy than fats are.

Finally, when you achieve ketosis, you may experience digestive symptoms like stomach pain. This is typical because you have removed something that your digestive system was used to. With this in mind, don't forget to take care of your gut health. Maintain intake of non-starchy veggies and foods that are high in fiber. If you are still concerned, you could talk to your doctor about a possible probiotic supplement.

Bad Breath

It may not sound appealing, but in the state of ketosis, you might experience bad breath. This is because ketones exit the body through urine AND breath.

Better Concentration

Finally! Another good symptom of being in ketosis is better concentration. Yes, initially you will experience headaches and clouded focus, but later on your mind will be clearer and your concentration and focus will be better than ever before.

Use Testing Strips

If you really want to be sure if you're in ketosis, you can buy a testing kit which you can use at home. Although instructions vary from manufacturer to manufacturer, the basic idea is testing strips which you saturate with urine.

Once you have the strip, you can saturate it with urine in two ways. The first is to hold the strip under your urine stream until it's saturated. The other method is to collect urine in a collecting cup and submerge the strip in it.

After saturating the strip, shake of the excess urine, wait for a few seconds (depending on package instructions), and correlate the color for results.

Can You Go on the Ketogenic Diet Forever?

This is a very, very important question. Let's say you have achieved ketosis and you have started losing weight; how long should you maintain the Ketogenic diet?

Remember that Keto is really a specialized diet, so we need more confirmatory studies to assess exactly how long it is safe to remain on this limited routine. Some people gained success within just 24 weeks of religiously following the rules, and some experts emphasize that you should not be on the Keto diet for longer than 12 months. But although opinions vary and we still don't have a specific cut off point for the diet, there are precautions which you ought to follow regardless. Always keep an eye on your kidney functions and hydrate whenever you feel thirsty.

Close monitoring is always essential while you're using Keto. If you decide to stop the Ketogenic diet, and are no longer under its strict rules, you can still maintain your weight (and health) by taking note of the following measures:

1. Make sure that you increase your carbs GRADUALLY. This means that you cannot binge on carbs just because you've decided that, okay, Keto time is over. Since you're counting carbs anyway, try to increase your carb intake by 10 grams daily for the first week and see how it goes.

2. Many experts say you must maintain a semblance of the low-carb diet, but no longer full Keto wherein your carbs are completely restricted. As a bridge, you could consider the low-carb paleo diet.

3. Still on the subject of carbs: when coming off the keto diet try to stay away from processed carbs.

4. Use tools to assess how many carbs you need now that you've lost weight. The BMR tool might help you here, but the best course of action is to always, always consult a doctor or a dietician if you have any doubts at all.

5. Now that you don't need to be on a high-fat diet, focus on your proteins. However, bear in mind that lean proteins are still best.

Remember that once you stop following the Keto diet, you may experience symptoms such as bloating or even weight gain. Don't panic. You are in a far better position now than before your diet, as you have already attained you ideal weight. All you need now is maintenance.

And guess what? Many people have demonstrated that they are able to maintain their health and ideal weight after coming off the Keto diet, simply by re-embracing a good old, well-balanced diet once more..

Key Takeaways

After you have reached your ideal weight though the Ketogenic diet, you can now try to maintain it using a slightly less-restrictive diet regimen. Remember to always prioritize your health. After all, losing weight is just the side effect of getting a healthy body from ketosis.

Chapter 10

Simple Keto Recipes

And now! We bring you 10 simple recipes that are keto-safe! We're making it even more exciting and easier since each of these recipes only has 5 ingredients – or less!

1. Low-Carb Chicken Nuggets

You may argue that you can buy chicken nuggets anytime, but let's be honest – we know that those frozen nuggets are processed and full of preservatives. So, why not try this recipe when you're craving chicken nuggets?

Ingredients:

2 cups of cooked chicken (you can also use left-over chicken)

1 tsp of garlic salt

8 oz of cream cheese

¼ cup of almond flour

1 medium-sized egg

Method: 1. Shred the chicken using an electric mixer; if you used left-over chicken, warm it up first before shredding.

2. When the chicken is shredded enough, add all the ingredients together and mix again using the mixer.

3. Once thoroughly combined, spoon the mixture in bite sized blobs onto a well-greased or lined baking tray.

4. Flatten the scooped mixture until you have the semblance of a nugget.

5. Bake for 12 to 15 minutes at 350 F, or until firm and golden.

2. Baked Dinner Sausage

Here's a quick fix when you're hungry for a tasty dinner. Aside from being very cheesy, it's also versatile in terms of ingredients.

Ingredients:

3 pounds of Italian sausage, turkey, chicken, or pork

8 ounces of mozzarella cheese

8 ounces of cream cheese

¼ cup of heavy cream

¼ cup of basil pesto

Method:1. Put the sausages in the casserole and bake in a pre-heated oven at 400 F for about half an hour.

2. While baking the sausages, mix the pesto, cream cheese, and heavy cream together for the sauce.

3. Spread the sauce on top of the baked sausage and top with mozzarella cheese.

4. Bake for another 10 minutes.

3. **Stuffed Pork Chops**

Pork chops are a classic Keto food and here's a recipe that puts an exciting twist on this reliable dish!

Ingredients:

2 to 2.5 ounces of thin cut, boneless pork chops (about 12)

8 ounces of provolone cheese (about 12 slices)

4 cloves of garlic

2.5 ounces of baby spinach

1 and ½ tsp of salt

Method:1. Prepare the rubbing mixture by pressing the garlic and combining it with salt.

2. Rub the mixture onto one side of the sliced chops. Place the chops on a baking sheet, rubbed side down.

3. Place spinach on top of the chop slices before adding the folded cheese.

4. Finally, top them with the second pork chop, this time with the rubbed side up.

5. Bake in a pre-heated oven at 350 F for 20 minutes before topping them with the rest of the folded cheese.

6. Bake again for another 10 to 15 minutes.

4. **Baked Eggs**

Here's another take on eggs – our favorite Keto-saver! It's super simple, too!

Ingredients:

3 ounces of ground pork or ground beef

2 ounces of shredded cheese

2 medium-sized eggs

Method:1. Place the ground meat on a baking sheet.

2. Form 2 holes in the ground meat, and crack the eggs into the holes.

3. Top the eggs with cheese.

4. Bake in the pre-heated oven at 400 F for about 10 to 15 minutes or until the eggs are done.

5. **Cheesy Meat Balls**

When you're craving meatballs, try this easy recipe!

Ingredients:

1 and ½ pounds of ground beef

4 ounces of mozzarella cheese

1 tbsp dried basil

2 pinches of pepper

2 tbsp of cold water

½ tsp salt

Method:1. In a bowl, combine the ground beef, pepper, basil, salt, and cold water. Mix well, using your hands or a wooden, spoon.

2. From the mixture, form about 10 patties.

3. Divide the cheese for the 10 patties.

4. Form a ball by wrapping the patty around the cheese.

5. Fry in butter until cooked or until the juices flow out.

6. **Smoked Salmon with Avocados**

This one is perhaps the easiest recipe, because there's no cooking required – you just need to assemble the ingredients!

Ingredients:

7 ounces of smoked salmon

½ cup mayonnaise

2 avocados

Salt and pepper

Method:1. Take the avocados and remove the pit. Using a spoon, scoop out the flesh and place on a plate.

2. Next, add the smoked salmon and a healthy scoop of mayo on the side.

3. Season with salt and pepper and enjoy!

7. **Mashed Cauliflower**

Are you craving mashed potatoes? Well, this is a great alternative!

Ingredients:

6 cups of chopped cauliflower heads

2 cloves of garlic, crushed

½ cup of chicken broth

1 bay leaf

1 tsp whole peppercorns

Method:1. Place the cauliflower in a saucepan and add enough water to cover. Bring to a boil.

2. When it's boiling, reduce heat and then simmer for another 10 minutes.

3. Drain and return to the saucepan.

4. In another small saucepan, add the remaining ingredients and bring to a boil before draining. Add salt if desired. Drain and discard the bay leaf, peppercorn, and garlic.

5. Add the broth to the cauliflower, mix and mash until you reach the desired consistency.

8. **Hot Chocolate**

From here on, we will be having Keto-safe drinks! We're starting with hot chocolate seeing that you might crave it when the weather is cold.

Ingredients:

6 ounces of sugar-free, high-quality chopped dark chocolate or chocolate chips

½ cup of heavy cream

½ cup of unsweetened almond milk

½ tsp vanilla extract

Method:1. Place almond milk and heavy cream in a saucepan, mix and heat until simmering. Remove from heat.

2. Add the vanilla extract and the chocolate. Whisk until the chocolate has melted and blended together with the cream and milk mixture.

3. Pour into an espresso cup and enjoy!

9. **Milkshake**

Another thing you might miss while on Keto is milkshake – so here's a great recipe to keep in mind!

Ingredients:

1 can, 13.5 ounce of coconut milk – discard coconut water and just retain the cream

¼ cup of allulose blend or Keto sweetener

1 cup heavy cream

2 tsp vanilla extract

2 cups of ice cubes

Method:1. Blend all the ingredients except ice in a blender until smooth.

2. Add the ice cubes and blend again until you reach shake consistency. Don't blend too much as it may make your shake too watery.

10. **Keto Tea Recipe**

Yes, we know that tea is accepted, but let's add a twist in your typical brewed tea.

Ingredients:

1 packet of tea

10 ounce of hot water

½ tbsp. MCT oil

½ tbsp. butter

Method:1. Steep the tea in the hot water according to packet instructions.

2. Combine tea, MCT oil, and butter in a blender and blend until smooth and creamy.

3. Serve and enjoy!

9 798748 188586